So You Want To Lose Weight But You Can't Stop Eating?

How to break free from the bondage of

food addiction and

stop the insanity of overeating.

With the Help and Power of God

You Too Can Be Set Free.

Written by Lacy Enderson

Author of ~ Addiction: A Personal Story

First printing December 2006

Bennett Deane Publishing
PO Box 630267
Simi Valley, CA 93063
Lacysjourney.com

ISBN: 978-0-6151-3791-9

Introduction

So you want to lose weight but you can't stop eating?

God knows I have lived that life before. I feel like I have a head full of valuable knowledge on how you too can stop overeating, yet putting it on paper is harder than you'd think. But I promise to give it my best try. If during the process I sound redundant and I repeat myself, I am trying to write down as much information in this book as possible so you may experience recovery from overeating and learn to live a life full of peace and freedom.

I know your plan is to discover a way to stop overeating and start losing weight and you acquired this book with immense excitement. Believe me, I understand. I bought more books and information than I can remember on how to lose weight. I was always bound and determined to find the one source of information that was going to free me forever from my food insanity. Problem, nothing ever provided the quick fix I was looking for. Nothing ever worked fast enough and I always found myself left discouraged and disappointed. The biggest problem of all was that I was seeking a way to lose weight when I needed to find the solution on how to quit eating. Weight wasn't my problem, eating was.

I know you want to lose weight or you wouldn't be reading this book. I know how disappointing it is to see that extra weight on your body day after day and have no idea how to get rid of it. I fully understand how it feels to wake up in the morning, vow a day of starvation, only to be gorging yourself with food within hours of your self proclaimed goal.

Didn't you know your body will not let you starve it? Our bodies are not capable of going hungry for very long. Eventually a binge is inevitable. Your body is on a timer. It knows when you need to eat. When you don't feed your body, it will let you know. You shouldn't think you can trick your system into submission. Your body is smarter than you think. And remember, starving yourself or depriving yourself of certain foods isn't the answer. Learning when to eat and eating for all the right reasons is. Since I am sure you have all heard that said before let me reassure you, I am not leaving you with just that information. But it is important that you understand that fact. Starvation is not the answer to your weight problem; learning when and how to eat right is.

The ultimate achievement is learning how to quit thinking about food so you can quit eating it. Most overeaters are obsessed with food. They wake up in the morning thinking about food and food is the last thought on their mind when they go to bed. For some of them, they wake up in the middle of the night thinking about food. For those who have a midnight food thought, they are probably also eating in the middle of the night. I have a friend who eats in her sleep. She wakes up in the morning to find empty boxes and wrappers where food used to be. Talk about an obsessive compulsive behavior? She has no control even while sleeping.

Imagine a day when the only reason thoughts of food cross your mind are because you are hungry? Imagine that you are grinding away at a busy task and your stomach growls. You say to yourself, oh yah, I haven't eaten yet. Maybe I should eat lunch? Imagine that day when the last thing on your mind is food and not only is there no time to think about food, you don't have time to eat it either? What a glorious day indeed. And it is possible. I know right now that thought is inconceivable. Believe me it can happen. It happened for me and it can happen for you. The best part is once you arrive the rest is easy. Upon your arrival there is no more hard work or effort. Sure there is self effort along the way but once the goal is achieved the rest is a piece of cake (well not exactly).

Just as countless others have given up alcohol or cigarettes and have gone days without obsessing over these substances, a food addict can be cured completely of food addiction. I know it is harder with food because we have to eat to stay alive but that obstacle becomes obsolete on our road to recovery. Imagine, recovering from food? I know it sounds silly but recovery is what we strive for.

Let me also mention I know what I am talking about when I say an alcoholic or a smoker can not only give up their substance addiction, but they can go days without thinking about them. I am a recovering alcoholic/smoker and I hardly ever think about smoking or drinking. Days go by without a single thought. One day you will discover that you too can go a whole day without thinking about overeating. You might think about food, but there is a difference. It is completely possible to think about food without eating it. That is when the real deliverance starts. Imagine a thought to eat that goes away as quickly as it enters your mind? The day of deliverance brings freedom from acting on every thought to eat. You will be delivered into the place where, if you don't need that food you won't eat it.

There is an important catch to mention. The way to recovery from any addiction in my opinion is through the help and the power of God. Now don't lose me here. I know some of you have a hard time with the concept of God. I do understand that. Not everyone has been blessed with an incredible relationship with God like the one I have. But you must try to understand, without

God's help it is almost impossible to be truly delivered from any substance or addiction. Sure there are those who can give up substance abuse by shear will power but it is not easy. In fact, it is downright difficult. If I can convince you that with God's help your success rate will quadruple will you at least be open-minded to the fact that there actually might be a God who wants to help you?

I promise I'll try not to get too preachy. I do enough of that in my book 'Addiction: A Personal Story.' I cannot fully instruct you on food recovery unless I am completely honest in telling you it is almost 100% the help and power of God. That is just the way it works. Nothing I ever tried before had any success rate compared to the deliverance I received when I let God take over. For those of you who have a hard time with the God thing I will share with you what was shared with me in the beginning of my quest. If you have a hard time believing in God, believe in my belief. Just get by on the fact that I believe that God is real and that He has been sent to help us. If you can at least believe in my belief, then you will have a starting point.

I don't want you to give up just because you are an atheist or an agnostic. I don't want you to become angry and rebellious at my mere suggestion that a belief in God is imperative. Admit it, stubborn rebellion never got you anywhere before and it won't do you any good here either. So get humble and get willing and let's seek to combat this life hindering food addiction. We are all in the same boat floundering around in a sea of despair. It is time to take the oars and row ourselves out of deep waters. It is time to set our feet on solid ground and experience life like God intended. So together let's go forward into a life full of peace and freedom. Come with me now and I will tell you how I did it.

Part 1 ~ In The Beginning

I grew up a skinny kid. In fact, to be honest, I have never had a weight problem a day in my life. Now don't close the book on me. I thought I had a weight problem. In fact most of my teen years were spent convinced I was fat. I was told I had a fat mind or a warped way of thinking. They said I looked in the mirror and saw myself as fat because I believed I was fat. I look back now and see I was never fat. I only thought I was fat. It was all in my mind. At that time my weight was the only thing I focused on. From the time I got up in the morning until the time I went to bed I thought about my weight. I was convinced, I was fat. I know now it was all in my mind. It was actually the only thing on my mind.

I wish I had a horrible devastating story to tell about how the people in my life caused me great distress and heartache. I wish I had stories to tell about situations that happened to me that ruined my life forever; you know the story about the uncle who crossed the boundaries? But there was none of that. We read about the obese middle aged woman who can't stop eating because she was molested as a child. Or the man who continuously eats because his father called him names and refused him love. That was not the case in my household. If it is a part of your past please don't think I am discounting your emotional problems as unimportant and please don't think I can't help you because I didn't go through the same devastating life events that you did. We all have different stories to tell and they are all equally important.

I think my first real food issue crept in at about the eighth grade. I was at my best friend's house one night for a slumber party and she introduced me to binging and purging. I didn't personally have a need to do this but she being a little overweight had been practicing this procedure for quite some time. Her mom had bought all kinds of donuts and pastries for the party. The kitchen was filled with every kind of imaginable party food. It was my favorite place to be, a party. And although I loved sweets I wasn't one to indulge in delicacies, I mean, even at the age of 13 I cared about what I looked like. But my friend told me I could eat all the donuts and ice cream I wanted and I could just throw them up when I was done. That way I never had to worry about gaining weight. That sounded like a good idea to me. So I did. I tried vomiting a few times throughout the evening. It didn't seem to be hurting me. I was actually excited to have learned this great method of eating anything I wanted and throwing it up.

And that was the way it all started. Just like that. I was an obsessive compulsive overeater and bulimic.

Within a few hours one evening I began a system of self destruction that would last me well into my young adult years. I began a bad habit that I would find very hard to break. I started down a road of pure misery. You know the saying; I sure wish I knew back then what I know today. It would have saved me years of buying and reading self help books on recovery from overeating like this one.

It amazes me how addictive some things are. I have heard it said that some people have an addictive personality and tend to become addicted to things more easily than others. That was me. I became addicted to bulimia. In fact, I became addicted to almost anything I could get my hands on throughout my life as I would soon discover. I confess I don't think it had much to do with weight in the beginning. I liked sweets and now I had a way of eating all of them I wanted without any worry of getting fat. But I wasn't already fat.

I became addicted to eating. I couldn't stop. It seemed all I thought about was food; how much I could get my hands on and into my mouth. The next thought was always where the closest bathroom was so I could get rid of it. Try hiding that from your parents for years.

I joined many activities in my teen years. I participated in school sports events, ran for school council, was involved in drama, public speaking, drill when I couldn't make up my mind who was more important to please; God, me or my boyfriend. Food became my comfort when I could not make a decision.

Food comforted me when I was confused. It comforted me when I knew my behavior disappointed my loved ones. When I was confused about my relationship I ate to distract me from guilt. And it was a funny thing; I didn't need to be eating in order to be distracted, just the thought of food was distraction enough to keep my mind off of my life and off my problems. If I was starving myself that day, then starvation was the distraction. The eating disorder was the mental focus that kept me from having to look at my life. Thinking about food or lack of it meant that I didn't have to think about anything else that was going on around me.

Food was the great escape from reality. My reality had become very uncomfortable and food allowed me to get my mind off the discomfort. I had circumstances in my life that I didn't like; aspects of my life I wanted to change that I couldn't change. Food fixed everything. Food substituted the decisions I just couldn't make. Food took the focus off the life events too difficult to live with so I wasn't plagued by my inability to do anything about them. I felt as a teenager I didn't have many rights and some things just weren't going to change for me no matter how bad I needed them to.

Part 2 ~ What Life Was Like

Thinking back over my life at all the crazy things I did to lose weight or recover from eating, I am amazed at my behavior. An eating disorder can be just as much a root of insane behavior as drug or alcohol addiction. I remember one day wanting to quit eating so bad that I put a piece of bologna and cheese separated by mayonnaise on my windowsill. I was in hopes as the food rotted and I ate it I would develop such a bad case of food poisoning that food would be the last thing I wanted for at least a few days. I was convinced that if I couldn't eat then I'd lose that extra few pounds and be on my way to happiness. I always thought if I were thin I'd be happy. Yet even when I was thin I was miserable. I learned it was all about my attitude to life that determined my happiness not what I looked like. Anyway the food never sat long enough to spoil. I ate it too soon. I am unsure if I'd actually have eaten it had it grown green mold; probably not.

One day I thought I'd take about six Contact cold pills all at one time. I knew six pills weren't enough to kill me. I thought maybe they'd make me just nauseous enough to keep me from eating. Sure the pills made my stomach sick but I was more alarmed by a constant ringing in my ears that lasted all day. I was actually with having boxes of candy around an obsessive overeater is an impossibility to get them sold without eating them. I managed to consume 56 boxes of M&M's on my own and owed the school that money out of my allowance. I remember lying in bed at night shoving gobs of M&M's in my mouth, one box after another. For some unknown reason I could not stop eating the candy. After a few nights of that insanity I gave the candy back. I refused to have it in my possession. Just as an alcoholic can't be around beer or a smoker around cigarettes, I couldn't be around food. If it was there, I ate it.

I grew quite accustomed to putting mustard on my lettuce and calling it a salad. I had learned mustard was very low in calories so I began putting it on everything. I stayed far away from mayonnaise and salad dressing because they were fattening but mustard on lettuce contained hardly any calories at all. Every now and then I'd go on some strange diet I had concocted that would lead me to my desired weight goal. I wish I could have understood the insanity of my behavior back then. I wish I had known about food and eating disorders yet they weren't discussed much when I was young. I might have taken a different approach rather than the one I had; compulsively overeating and then starving or throwing up to get the extra weight off.

When I was younger losing the weight never

seemed to be a problem for me. I could get the weight off. It was keeping it off I couldn't do. I ate for such strange reasons; fear, intimidation, anger, imperfection, changes that wouldn't take place, people who wouldn't do it my way, impatience; life took to long. I needed life to change yesterday but nothing important to me ever happened fast enough. I just didn't understand the insanity of what I was doing when I was young. I was eating to drown out uncomfortable feelings but as a teenager I didn't know that was the reason.

I remember one diet I tried that seemed to work well for me. I ate a half a carrot in the morning before I left the house. I ate an apple for lunch and I'd finish the carrot when I returned home from school. I'd eat a normal dinner, whatever my mom cooked, and I'd go out and run around the block a few times each night. I didn't allow myself any treats so I didn't have to worry about overeating them. I only allowed myself these given foods at those given times. But it was never long before a catastrophe would pop up in my life and I'd be back to consuming Ding Dongs and Twinkies in hopes of feeling better. I didn't know how to deal with uncomfortable feelings. I always wanted to fix them. I couldn't stand imperfection or people out of control. Any part of my life that was out of order or a nasty person who intimidated me was a reason to compulsively overeat.

I want to talk about intimidating people for a moment. I was very concerned with what people thought about me. I wanted everybody to like and accept me always. I didn't like it when I thought someone was angry with me or upset about something I did. I felt extremely uncomfortable with the tension surrounding angry people. I was always very sensitive. I tended to feel responsible for other peoples bad moods. I always felt I was somehow to blame. If someone was in a bad mood I always assumed they were mad at me. If I was certain that it wasn't about me I would set out on a mission to make the moody person feel better. This was really just an attempt to make myself feel better. But if I tried to help an angry person and they wouldn't accept my help I instantly became defensive and turned the whole situation around to be about me.

Becoming angry at an angry person meant I wasn't required to feel compassion towards them or try to help because now my anger was more important. Because I was so self absorbed I honestly didn't have time to care about others on a deeper level. My concern was surface level and shallow; how did it affect me. See, it really didn't matter to me why an angry person was having a bad day, for my well being they just needed to stop. I was good at being a victim. I felt sorry for myself and I wanted everyone else to feel sorry for me too. I could manipulate any situation to get the focus on me and I was good at it.

It wasn't until I got older that I realized other peoples bad moods are not always my fault. And people are allowed to be in a bad mood without my taking it personally and trying to fix it. I found that when I tried to mend another person I only made matters worse anyway because my heart wasn't right. My motives and intent were wrong and selfish. I always managed to do more damage than good. There is a saying that hurting people hurt other people. I guess that is what I did for a long time.

Feeling responsible for another person's bad day led me to food. The anxiety I felt being around an angry person made me desire food. I did not know how to separate my feelings from another person's anger. I couldn't allow them to feel their own feelings. I wanted to control and manipulate the situation. Anger, rage, sadness and depression in others were unacceptable to me and too uncomfortable for me to deal with. Food was a great solace; especially once I became the victim. I could go to the local Bob's Big Boy eat a plate of Spaghetti and Chili and a huge Hot Fudge Sundae cake and completely escape uncomfortable feelings. I would have my own private pity party; poor me.

Did you know that people can have a bad day, yell, scream, holler, cry and act crazy and it could have nothing to do with you? Did you know that a loved ones break down is not the time for your self pity? Didn't you know that you are not the most important person in the world and that other people do have legit reasons for having bad days that are absolutely not nor should they be about you? You are not the center of the universe and the world does not revolve around you.

I have learned that it is OK if someone is upset with me. I am not God. I will make mistakes. Even during those times when someone is upset with me for something I didn't do, it is OK. People are allowed to react in any manner they see fit. Life cannot always be about me. I cannot always control and dictate my surroundings. I must let other people be who they are. If they want to have a bad day then so be it. It is not always about what I want or what I'm comfortable with.

There is freedom in allowing other people to live their own lives. We might not like or feel comfortable with their choices but it is Ok to accept them as they are, bad choices and all. I have learned it is easier to accept uncomfortable angry people if I am sympathetic towards them. If I try to consider there might be an underlying reason for the cantankerous or foul mood it is easier to accept the negative emotions. People need empathy. They need someone who cares. If I am always so concerned about myself and how other people are making me feel I will never be the compassionate soul I should be.

I can't help others if I am always focused on myself. Once we take our eyes off of ourselves and truly care about what another person is going through our need to eat will subside. We will no longer have a need to escape uncomfortable feelings because angry people will no longer intimidate us and make us feel uncomfortable. When we quit looking in a mirror at ourselves and look outward at others we will be more compelled to see their needs and not our own. As we quit focusing on our problems and start caring about others we will have less reason to eat. Our problems will begin to fade in comparison to what other people go through and instead of seeking our own personal comfort we will seek how we can be of help to someone else.

One day when my daughter was ten she took an ice cream sandwich out of the freezer at eight in the morning and ate it for breakfast. After she finished the first she asked if she could have another one. I asked her what was wrong. I asked her what was troubling her. She said she had been given permission to spend a certain amount of her allowance at the local carnival but she had spent the whole thing. She was afraid her father would be mad at her. She ate because she feared her father's reaction. The ice cream was her comfort.

I am sure you've heard of comfort foods. Those are

the foods we choose that make us feel better. And to be honest there isn't anything wrong with comfort foods in moderation. But it's the moderation that is near impossible for the compulsive overeater. Each ice cream is an attempt to make the discomfort go away but when it doesn't more food is needed. As the food is being eaten the remorse sets in. Everyone who eats excessively for any given length of time feels badly in the end. For those who binge and purge they just get rid of the vast amount of eaten food. If they are lucky they can end the insanity but most overeaters look at the vomiting as a time to start over; and the cycle continues.

Exercise was a big part of my weight reduction plan. I learned that if I ran in the morning before school, ran during track, walked to and from school and rode my bike in the afternoon I could not only lose weight I could tone my body until I looked like I wanted to. Becoming addicted to exercise became just as debilitating and life hindering as any other addiction. Instead of keeping fit for my heart and my mental well being I was going to the gym, running, walking and riding my bike as another mental distraction from those situations in my life I could not control. Exercise became another bondage that had me bound.

Jumping ahead into the present concerning exercise, for over ten years I refused to exercise. After my deliverance I was never going back into that bondage again. Today I have learned to exercise for all the right reasons. I am in my forties and I was told by the doctor that exercising was good for my heart and also helped lower my cholesterol. I also know that if I walk on my treadmill for at least twenty minutes each day I can eat a sweet treat at night. It is a fair payoff and one that works well for me.

When I was in college I had an apartment two miles from school. I also had a car. But I refused to drive the car. I walked everywhere I went. I got up in the morning extra early so I could go running. I walked the two miles to and from school. I then ran more after school. College was a hard time for me. For one I had a roommate that wasn't perfect enough for my lifestyle. She didn't keep the bathroom clean enough and that drove me crazy. She could not live up to my high expectations because they were so high even I couldn't reach them.

I started smoking during the first few days of college and that started a whole new chain of self destruction. As my body craved cigarettes I found myself eating more. I hated smoking so I ate. I hated eating so I smoked. I was very disappointed in myself for allowing myself to start smoking. But once I became addicted to nicotine and found I was thinking about the cigarettes as much as I thought about food, I was a mess. Do I eat or do I smoke?

An addiction is an addiction. Eating disorders can be just as debilitating for the overeater as alcohol is for the alcoholic. No addiction is worse than another to the one who suffers. For a person who uses a substance to escape from life it soon becomes apparent that any addiction will do. I was an emotional and mental mess and I was addicted to anything that allowed me a moment's peace of mind. Even though it became obvious that the peace of mind I experienced was a false and temporary perception.

For example, when I was in college I felt lonely and stressed out. I left a boyfriend back at home three hours away. The relationship was not a very good one and deep down inside I knew I needed to use the time away to end our association but that was hard for me. He called all the time and came on weekends to visit. It was easier for me to stay in the relationship. But the inner turmoil of knowing I was making the wrong decision was overwhelmingly difficult to deal with so I ate.

I would make an entire sheet of toll house chocolate chip cookies, eat the whole batch and then throw them up. During the process of making the cookies, eating the cookies and then getting rid of the cookies I put myself into another world that did not allow difficult decisions or uncomfortable feelings. For the time it took to complete the cookie process I was not required to think about the relationship. I thought about the cookies. That was my temporary time of peace; false peace yet peace nonetheless.

I remember holiday times when friends would give me boxes of Sees candy. I loved Sees candy yet was very aware that I could not have entire boxes of candy around me. Just like gallons of ice cream in the freezer were definitely not allowed. Of course I would eat the candy, one piece after another. Of course the entire time I put those chocolate morsels in my mouth I was telling myself, "This will be your last one." I was never able to stop.

I discovered this great defense against boxes of chocolates in my presence. I would eat a few and then spray the rest of the chocolate with Lysol. I knew if I put the box in the trash I'd dig it up. But if I sprayed it first with chemicals I wouldn't bother. Sometimes I needed an extra measure of self will and help. Sometimes it was about whatever worked. Spraying the chocolate with Lysol worked for me.

Another one of my fond memories was the time I bought a book called, "Feeding the Hungry Heart." It was a very good book and I enjoyed reading it. This book taught me how I ate to fill the empty hole in my heart. I ate because I lacked love. I ate because I needed intimacy and affection. I ate for all the wrong reasons. I'd climb into bed at night with that book and a bag of popcorn or M&M's and I would proceed to eat my way right through the reading of that book. I needed help but I hadn't found it yet. I was on my way but I hadn't arrived. I figured I was going to eat anyway. So reading while I ate served a good purpose. I could attempt to eat all my problems away while reading self help books on how I could potentially stop such insane behavior. Talk about an oxy moron.

I ate a lot when I was lonely. I have been married three times. After my first husband left me I became a single mother of three small children. I wasn't used to being alone. It was not easy for me. I was constantly searching for a new man to replace the one I lost. I wanted a man and I wanted him now. Because a man wasn't available when I needed one I ate to fill the void. But it wasn't just eating out of boredom; I was literally trying to fill a hole in my heart. Needless to say it was futile eating. It never solved anything. At the end of the food there was still a huge hole in my heart.

There was a hole in my heart for a long time. I tried filling it with food, cigarettes, alcohol, relationships and anything else I could find that offered me a quick fix. But nothing ever worked long enough. All of my remedies offered temporary relief. I was always right back where I started from, lost and lonely and filled with inner struggles. Problems consumed my life and I felt responsible for fixing every one of them. I lived in the moment. I needed everything better right now. I had no concept of maybe tomorrow. If the problem wasn't solved right now I became insane. That is why I ate.

I remember nights when I'd be all alone. The kids would be sleeping and I'd be on the phone for hours with my best friend. Because she wasn't satisfying the intimacy I needed I'd look for a substance to help me feel better. I remember thinking, food has too many calories, and alcohol does too, so I'd decide to smoke cigarettes instead. The problem was I never had any cigarettes available. At this time in my life I was not a daily smoker. I smoked occasionally when I'd have a drink. So I'd walk up and down the sidewalk looking for other peoples cigarette butts. Talk about desperation. I was an emotional wreck.

The inner conflict of needing a solution now kept me in a constant state of frenzy. The food offered immediate satisfaction therefore is was desirable. The pleasant taste of the food presented a positive experience that for a moment pushed the negative feelings out. Our senses respond to pleasure. I believe there is a chemical reaction in the brain which gives off a pleasure signal when good food is consumed. I don't know that for certain but I think I have read that somewhere. When problems consumed me and they were all I could think about I had to replace the negative thinking with positive thoughts. Not knowing any other way, I ate. Thus the pleasure of the food overrode the overwhelming burden of the problem; unfortunately only for the moment.

It wasn't until I became pregnant at the age of eighteen that I was delivered from bulimia. Having another more important person to think about actually took my eyes and mind off of me. I found myself so involved in this baby inside of me I thought less and less about food. I now had a healthy distraction. It also helped that I had morning sickness for the first six months of my pregnancy. I weighed less after my baby was born than before I got pregnant. Of course food insanity returned after the pregnancy but I was completely delivered from bulimia never to binge and purge again. Habits are hard to break but given enough time they can be undone. Nine months of pregnancy was the time I needed to break the bulimia habit. I refused to go back to that miserable existence for anything in the world. I was just grateful to have a baby to occupy my thinking.

I need to mention that some people suffer from personality disorders, depression topping the list. I believe people suffer from chemical imbalances in their brains which dictate certain behaviors. I know that some people experience inner rage and anger due to brain malfunction. I do understand that sometimes those who suffer can't find relief. Substance abuse has proven to be higher among those who are plagued with certain personality and anxiety disorders. It is important for those who have rage or depression or those who just don't feel right to seek medical help. Food can be a great comfort for the depressed but better yet would be some therapy or possibly medication. Everyone is different and unique to their own dilemma. It is important to discover what your personal struggle stems from; addiction, an underlying medical problem, or both.

Part 3 ~ What Life Is Like Now

Food addiction is a serious matter especially for the extremely overweight and the obese. A lot of extra weight on a person is bad for the heart. Extra weight can lead to metabolic syndrome disease and possible diabetes. Being overweight is not only hard on the body it is damaging to self esteem. An overweight person gets stared at, made fun of and judged. I don't know how many times I have heard some unsympathetic person judge the overweight for eating ice cream or eating at all. I wish everyone knew just how hard it is for overweight people. People need to understand that heavy people would love to be thin. Why wouldn't they? If an overweight person could find the miracle needed to lose the weight I guarantee they would take it. It's not that easy. Losing weight for the food addict is extremely difficult. It's not always their fault. A little care and concern would do a lot more good than judgment and criticism.

Addiction usually starts in the mind. A thought becomes an obsession and the obsession turns into a compulsion. The compulsion turns into a habit and off we go. Habits are hard to break but can be broken if enough time is given to undoing the mental process. As we replace the obsessive thought with another thought eventually we break the cycle of food obsession. For example, instead of thinking about a cookie one could call a friend on the phone and ask her how she's doing. Not that eating a cookie is wrong but if you've already had a few and you're craving more because you can't pay your gas bill change you're thinking. Learning to change the way we think takes us off the road of insanity and puts us onto the road of recovery.

Remember in the beginning when I told you that this road to recovery has a higher success rate with the power and help of God? Well, this is where He comes in. Since we've already established the fact that there is a God or at least that I believe in God, and we've accepted a willingness to let Him help us, I'm just going to continue based on that. We've prayed and asked God for the willingness to make us willing. Using the first three steps of the twelve step recovery program we will build a foundation; first we admitted we are powerless over food and that our lives had become unmanageable, we came to believe in a power greater than ourselves that could restore us to sanity, and we made a decision to turn our will and our lives over to the care of God. We are basically going to exchange our food addiction, our reliance on the comforting affects of food to help us feel better, for an addiction to God or a new dependence on Him.

I always believed in God. From first grade on I attended church. I went to Sunday school every Sunday; I attended church events on Wednesdays and Fridays. I went to summer and winter church camps every year from fourth grade until I graduated High School. Believing in God was never a problem. I knew there was a God. It was almost as if God enabled me to know Him. I don't remember anything profound ever happening that would lead me to believe in Him. I never witnessed any big miracles or His physical presence. I just knew he existed. I guess I am one of the more fortunate ones. I hear it isn't like that for all people. Believing in God is a struggle for some and for others they never find Him. I am challenging you if you don't know God, start today by asking Him to reveal Himself to you. Everyday as you work towards food recovery ask Him to manifest Himself in your life. If you truly seek Him you will find Him.

Some of you were raised to believe that God was judgmental and condemning. You were brought up fearing the wrath of God. You chose along time ago that God wasn't worthy of your relationship with Him and you shunned Him from your life. Over the years I have witnessed God's goodness and grace in my life many times. I have seen the hand of God working in my circumstances in powerful ways. Maybe that reality makes it easier for me to see Him as a loving God but as

He begins working in your life also you too will see Him in a new and different light.

I have no doubt that God loves me completely and crowns me with His compassion. God understands. He is patient, long suffering, he cares about everything I go through. He doesn't say I will never have troubles what he says is he will walk with me and help me through each and every one of them. God is gentle, he is kind and he is most of all loving. Begin this day to change the way you think about God. If you are going to seek out His help you must first believe He wants to help you. God does not play favorites. What He has done for me He will do for you. Humbly submit yourself to His will and He will deliver you. God's ultimate desire is to see people delivered. Accept His peace and freedom today and begin to walk in newness of life.

For many people including myself it is easy to think that God doesn't love us. We look back over our lives at all the terrible things we've done and we can't imagine how God could possibly love and forgive us. It is easy to fall into that trap of self condemnation. I know for years I struggled to receive God's forgiveness. Although I realize now it wasn't so much God's forgiveness I needed but my own. I held myself in contempt for along time because of the wrong I had done and the lives I had damaged.

Self centered people tend to hurt others. Maybe we don't mean to but we do none the less. Learning to forgive ourselves is important. Realizing that God's forgiveness is eternal is crucial to our mental well being. There is nothing we have ever done that will make God love us any more or any less than He does right now. We are told if we confess our sins God will forgive us. Holding on to guilt is futile. We believe a lie when we tell ourselves God couldn't possibly love or forgive us. It is time to let that deception go. Turn it over to God and ask Him to help you receive forgiveness, not only from Him but from yourself also.

Apologizing to those we hurt is critical to our recovery. Being sorry sets us free from the guilt that leads us to food. I know as stubborn and rebellious people we tend to have a need to be right. We kick and scream to get our own way. Letting go of the need to be right is of vital importance. It is OK to be wrong even if you are not. Believe me, you will feel better and come out the winner in the end. I know that is against everything you've been taught. It doesn't matter. Your peace and freedom is far more important than being right. Believe me. I know what I am talking about.

I know that if I have harmed someone and they are angry with me I feel uncomfortable. Because discomfort leads to eating I will eat because I feel bad for what I have done. If I apologize then I release myself from the feelings of guilt. I no longer eat to feel better because I have let go of the burden of the guilt that makes me feel bad.

It is wise to remember that we are not responsible for another person's response to our apology. Not everyone is going to accept that we are sorry. It is not as important to our recovery how people respond. We can only do our part and allow others to do theirs. Of course we want our apology to be accepted but we can't control that nor should we try. If we attempt to force an obstinate person to accept our apology now we've created another problem; anger, defensiveness and control issues. We say we are sorry, we mean it, we do our best to make the situation right, and then we walk away with peace and freedom.

As I mentioned before, believing in God was never my problem, but trusting in Him was a different matter. Knowing God and trusting God were two different issues. They were not the same. Trusting in God meant that I believed He could solve all of my problems. Trusting that God could solve my problems meant that I reached for God during discomfort and not food. Turning my will and my life over to God meant I had to believe He was smarter than I was and could make better decisions than I could. It was easy to wake up in the morning and turn my life over to the care of God but actually leaving my life there was difficult. How could I really trust that God was going to work out my problems? If I couldn't see Him working how was I suppose to believe that He was?

You've heard it said before, practice makes perfect. As I practiced this principle and experienced God working to solve my problems it became easier each time to trust Him again. As I continued reaching for God instead of food I slowly lost my dependence on food and developed a new dependence on God. (Note: Sometimes you will have to wait. God's timing is not always the same as ours. But don't give up. Keep trusting no matter what.) God started doing for me what I could not do for myself. Now I actually wake up in the morning excited to see what God is going to do next. Developing a constant contact with God is of vital importance. Every single day you must practice praying to Him. As you talk to God your relationship with Him will grow. As you get closer to God and your belief in Him strengthens, trusting in Him will get easier.

For example; years ago my husband and I fell into some unfortunate financial problems. Because we didn't have the money to pay the bills we were evicted from our home. For thirty days I knew I'd have to pack and leave the home I'd lived in for years. I had absolutely no idea where I'd be going. This was a very disturbing time for me. If I had eaten a gallon of ice cream to ease my discomfort at the end of the gallon I'd still be suffering the mental anguish of the problem I had no control over. Instead of eating the ice cream I prayed and asked God to fix the problem. Each day upon awakening I thanked God for solving the problem. Even when I couldn't see any change I still thanked Him. At the end of the thirty days He provided us with a temporary place to stay and a new home to live in two weeks later.

Even though we had been evicted and our credit was bad, the new landlady said she didn't care. She said she had a gut feeling that we would make good tenants and she let us rent her house. That was a work of God. God spoke to the landlady's heart and told her to let us rent her home and she did. Now, if I had eaten the gallon of ice cream and each day there after piled food into my mouth while I cried and whined about how bad my life was the circumstances probably would have ended with a far worse outcome. Taking the problem to God and allowing Him to work it out for me provided a much favorable result.

I am not saying that turning your problems over to God will always offer instantaneous total relief. You might actually have to turn them over and over again throughout the next few days or even weeks. Over time as you practice this principle the relief will come quicker.

You might not experience a huge deliverance overnight from life's burdens. But giving them to God will sure lighten the load. As your load lightens and the burdens diminish focusing on God and His answers becomes easier. As your focus on God gets clearer and you begin looking to Him instead of the problems, the problems begin to fade in comparison to the hope that develops within. As a new hope springs up within you an overwhelming excitement takes over and you will find that no problem can get you down. We begin to look at problems as opportunities to see God work. I am not saying you will welcome problems but they will begin taking on a whole new meaning. As the uncomfortable feelings of fear and anxiety decrease your need to eat will also.

Developing the trust you need truly enables you to walk in peace and freedom. But you must spend time with God in order to develop that trust. Even those who have been trusting in God for years require daily time with God to renew their relationship. What I'm saying is, not one time in all of my life did food ever solve a problem; ever, but I have experienced countless times where God has. So looking at the facts, why turn to food when the end result is always the same; feelings of shame, remorse and failure, when you can turn to God who is standing right outside your heart waiting for you to ask Him in.

Doubt and unbelief have a way of creeping in no matter how hard we try to trust in God's provision. I think it's just human nature to worry. Even after years of giving God my problems and experiencing positive outcomes, when there is a catastrophe I tend to react. Now granted my reaction is far less dramatic than it used to be. I don't freak out and get all excited anymore. Today I might take my prayer into the bathroom where I can be alone with God and let Him know how I feel. God wants to talk with us. He wants to be our friend. I've been known to spend quite a while in the bathroom praying until I felt better. But I always felt better knowing I was giving my problems to a God who truly does care and who really does help and not to a box of cookies. There is comfort in knowing that.

The alternative to spending alone time with God is going to the freezer. If I am presented with a devastating situation I can't control; you know those tragedies of life you can't do anything about, and I go to food instead of God I am basically hiding under the problem. I am not doing anything to get rid of the problem. The problem remains right there before me when I've finished eating.

For example, If you've received one of those door hangers that lets you know your water bill wasn't paid and your water will be shut off in five days don't go to the cupboard. Not one cookie, not one Ding Dong is going to pay that water bill. And maybe God isn't going to pay the water bill either but I guarantee you this, if you take that water bill and present it to God you have just gotten rid of the burden of it. Eating a box of Twinkies increases the burden. You don't have to carry around the burden of an unpaid bill anymore. If you've done all you can and you still can't pay the bill thank God that He is bigger than your uncomfortable situation and go read a good magazine. No sense in eating away something that isn't going to leave. Start thanking God for all of the great things he has done for you. Change your thinking so you're not focused on the problem. Focus on other solutions God has already provided.

Try to remember a time from the past when you were in dire straights and everything worked out just fine. Dwell on that thought. Soon you'll be wondering why you ever wasted so much time worrying. God is a big God. He is bigger than every single one of your problems. He might not answer you the way you'd like Him to but give Him time and He'll answer you with a plan that will work better than any plan you had in mind. You see God doesn't work on the same schedule as we do. He isn't limited by time and space. His ways are higher than our ways. He isn't shocked by our problems. He sees right past the complaint to the solution. Thank Him in advance for having all the answers. Thank Him in advance for knowing exactly what to do. You begin to develop a new mindset. It is a mindset that works. It is a way of thinking that brings peace and freedom and that is what we strive for.

I've been told before that God doesn't need my help. I've been told to get out of His way so He can work. I do believe that sometimes there are things we can do to rectify a problem. It is important to ask God for divine direction. Ask Him if there is something you can do. Tell Him you are willing and able to do whatever he suggests. He will use people, places and things to reveal to you what you can do to help. Maybe someone will call with an unexpected job or a financial gift. Maybe it will be nothing more than an abundance of peace that calms your heart and mind. Be willing and open and then watch how God works. You will be amazed.

God is creative. He can and does help in remarkable ways. I have found that if I am constantly open to hear His voice He will reveal His plans to me. If I actively seek His perfect will, it will be found. Remain willing and able. But still remember to get out of His way. Our impatience can ruin everything. If we take matters into our own hands due to desperation the end result could be worse than the initial problem. We have to be able to wait for God's timing. Ask God for direction. Give

Him the situation and let it go.

God is in control. If you gave Him the problem, believe it is taken care of. Every time the problem creeps back into your mind immediately say, "God is in control. It is taken care of." The goal here is to get the problem off your mind. Problems lead overeaters to food. Problems are real but dwelling on them is good for nothing. We have to believe that a power greater than ourselves can handle every problem in our life. A great cliché to learn is, "Let go, let God."

Someone once suggested writing each problem on a piece of paper and putting it in what is called a God box. Once the problem is placed in the box the goal is to leave it there. We pray about the problem. We ask God to fix it for us. We thank Him for being a big God; bigger than the problem and then we put it in the box. People have told me that later on when they open the box to remind themselves of past problems they couldn't even remember some of the problems they had previously written down. At the time when they wrote the problem on the paper those problems were huge and devastating. Now they were not only solved but forgotten.

Another approach that works well is finding someone who suffers similar problems as yours and praying for them. When my children were younger and I was going through my second divorce I found myself lost in a world of confusion. I had no idea what to do and I was consumed with thoughts of self destruction and impending doom. I could not get my mind off myself for anything. I sat in my garage for hours eating candy, one piece after another, waiting for some miracle from God to rescue me from my horrible dilemma.

My boys played baseball with a local pastor's son and during the games I'd tell the pastor all about my personal woes. I feel sorry for him now when I think back because he probably got real tired of me always approaching him with my problems. He would tell me to find someone else going through a similar situation and pray for that person. It sounded like a good idea but was very difficult. I just couldn't seem to get my mind off myself long enough to care about someone else. But with time and practice I actually found myself sharing my time with others who were also suffering from troubling situations. It wasn't that my life all of a sudden got better; it was that I stopped thinking so much about my life.

As I quit dwelling on myself and started helping others I felt better. When I wasn't so focused on me and how bad I thought my life was I ate less. I wasn't consumed with grief piling food in my mouth in an attempt to feel better. I made sure that every time my mind turned towards myself I prayed about it and then went into prayer for another person.

Praying for someone else provided mental relief. Mental relief meant less anxiety and worry. Part of the recovery process is to get rid of self pity. Helping others takes our minds off ourselves and self pity begins to disappear. When I took my mind off of myself and seriously started caring for others I ate less, I felt better, I was less self consumed and I didn't need food to quench my discomfort. The discomfort started diminishing all on its own.

One of the more important steps in the 12 step recovery program is taking a personal inventory of ourselves and admitting our wrongs to ourselves to God and to someone else. Since I have already mentioned apologizing to others and giving up our right to be right, we've already discussed the first part of this process. But there is also the part where we write down on paper the exact nature of these wrongs and tell someone. We are only as sick as our secrets. For some of us we have committed some hefty crimes against others. We have offended others in ways we wouldn't want anyone to know about. Unfortunately these hidden secrets lead overeaters to food. As difficult as it sounds there is a freedom that comes from getting these secrets out that is far more rewarding than any shame you might feel. I promise you, if you can truly be honest with yourself and someone else you will experience a peace like you have never felt before. It is as if the whole world lifts off your shoulders and you no longer have to carry around that extra baggage ever again.

This is a principle that has been helping addicts for years. If it didn't work they wouldn't require it. It works. It works well. During your recovery process begin making a list of all those people you have harmed. Then make a list of all those people who have harmed you. When you find yourself eating uncontrollably ask yourself if it has anything to do with another person; if it does put that person on your list. Each day God will reveal more and more to you as you are willing to find freedom from these offenses and resentments. As you put them down on paper you are getting them out of your head. As these negative thoughts and feelings are removed from your thinking you will be better capable of thinking right thoughts. Right thinking leads to peace and freedom; the goal we are moving towards.

I highly encourage support group participation. There is nothing more encouraging than camaraderie with others going through the same thing we are. A group also gives us something else to focus on. I know from experience that members of groups also go out to coffee or dinner. Many attend dances and conventions. I have many very dear friends from support groups who gather together occasionally to do something out of the ordinary. It is a good idea to get new friends who are also trying to overcome food addiction. In recovery nothing changes if nothing changes. Change is an important part of our growth.

If you find eating at night the biggest problem schedule a meeting or a movie at night. If the morning hour is most difficult find a morning meeting and then go out to coffee. I found the hardest part of the day for me was at 3:30 in the afternoon when the last soap opera aired. I started watching soaps in the morning and they kept me occupied all afternoon. When they ended I was absolutely lost. It was that time from 3:30 until bed that was the hardest part of the day for me. I found that after dinner meetings or a movie helped me the most. If you have children and you feel house bound, take them to the park or to the McDonald's play land. Find out what your triggers are. Learn to be aware of the time of day when you are most likely to eat. Be encouraged, it won't be like that forever. As soon as the eating habit is broken you will find these times aren't triggers anymore. Just be prepared in the beginning. The start of any new resolution is always the hardest.

It will get to the point when the triggers will become less and less. Soon you'll be staring at the mountains thinking about how beautiful the trees are;

you won't be thinking about food wishing you had some chocolate to fill the empty space. There won't be an empty space because God's love will be in there. There won't be a bad time of day because everyday all day long will be glorious and worth living. Life will take on a whole new meaning. When problems come up your spiritual defense against them will be so strong maybe for a second you'll be caught off guard but then you'll take that problem and give it to God where it belongs. You will get so good at this you'll be smiling and content and people will want to know what drugs you are on.

Before I close I must talk about recovery's number one saboteur: relationships. I have known of well meaning men and women in sobriety who go back to drinking because of a bad relationship. I have seen people free from nicotine for years start smoking again because of a quarrelsome relationship and I have seen overweight people gorging themselves on food because someone in their life whom they thought loved them left them feeling afraid and anxious. Relationships in my opinion are the number one killer of all recovery. So what do we do about it? You guessed right, we give our relationships to God. And we don't take them back no matter what.

People will disappoint us. They will hurt us. They will leave us. Who cares? We are far more important and valuable than what another person thinks of us. In fact, we are precious commodities to be cherished and if someone isn't cherishing us they don't deserve us anyway. Now I am not advocating divorce. I believe if couples really try they can make any relationship work. What I am saying is food is not going to make your husband faithful. Food is not going to make your wife pay attention to you. Food is not going to stop the verbal or physical abuse. It's just not going to happen so don't eat your heartache away.

Take the problem to God. Don't yell and scream and get in an uproar. That is not going to fix your unhealthy relationship. Take the situation to God. Go in the bathroom and tell God how you feel. Ask God to share with your partner how you feel. God will tell your other half what needs to be heard. You don't have to say a word. Your complaint will only invite anger and angry people don't listen anyway. Angry people are so involved with themselves instead of listening as they should; they are planning what they are going to say next. I am serious when I say; for the sake of your recovery learn to bite your tongue. For your own good, practice keeping your mouth shut.

Because I do feel that communication in a relationship is important if what you need to say must be said give it some time so you can calm down. Wait a few hours or even days if need be so your emotional level is lower. A calm attitude will produce better results. The goal here is not to set up a situation where you are eating food uncontrollably because someone upset you or hurt your feelings. You will find that your emotional well being is far more important than making sure your loved one knows exactly how you feel. You will discover that making yourself heard all the time is just not that important.

Addicts need to learn conflict avoidance at all cost. I was told in alcoholics anonymous that anger was not a luxury I could afford. Well I feel the same is true for the food addict. If you are in a situation where another person's actions are making you crazy, leave the room. Pray, cry, even think an occasional bad thought but then thank God for being in control. Thank Him for taking care of the problem. Thank Him for peace and freedom and find something to do that makes you happy. If you are caught in a situation you absolutely can't do anything to change, let it go.

Be careful that you are not picking a fight on purpose to give you a reason to binge. As an alcoholic I used to start fights so I'd have an excuse to drink. Addicts can become addicted to chaos. We are not used to peace so if life becomes too peaceful and serene we will sabotage it by causing an argument. I know this seems ridiculous but it happens all the time. If you find yourself creating disturbances because life is getting too good, be aware. Awareness is the first step to changing irrational behavior. This behavior has to be smashed. In recovery you must learn how to take care of yourself, spiritually, emotionally, mentally and physically. The first step is admitting you are powerless not only over food but over people, places and things also. But remember and be reassured, God has all power.

Begin today changing the way you think about yourself. Practice daily affirmations. Instead of calling yourself a failure refer to yourself as a work in progress. We are told our recovery is based on progress not perfection. No one is perfect except for God so don't beat yourself up if you fall down. Get right back up and begin again. Begin today by seeing yourself the way God sees you. Remember God made you in His own image and He doesn't make mistakes. Start believing in yourself the way God does.

Look forward to the end result. Be grateful for where you are going not discouraged at where you have been. There is nothing you can do to change the past. It is now up to you to close the door on what cannot be changed and walk forward into the future God has prepared for you. Life is full of ups and downs and every now and then a curve ball will get thrown your way. If you stay strong and stand your ground there is nothing you can't overcome. With your new attitude and God's help nothing will ever be too difficult again. You will do all things through Christ who gives you strength and with God's help you will recover from overeating and food addiction. You will discover and receive the peace and freedom God so graciously gives.

Part 4 ~ In Conclusion

God is always in control.

God can do for you what you can't do for yourself.

God loves you no matter what.

God has even your most difficult situations taken care of.

God cares deeply for you.

God wants you to give your problems to Him.

God wants you to quit focusing on yourself and begin to see the beauty all around you.

God wants you to cherish yourself.

God wants you to require others to cherish you.

God would rather see you come to Him in tears than anger. Anger destroys. Tears are of humble submission. Humbly submitting yourself to God and His will lifts you up.

God is working on your behalf even when you don't see Him.

God knows exactly what you need.

God is all you need.

God is bigger than all your fears.

God is greater than all your struggles.

God provides lasting comfort.

God gives peace and freedom and a whole new way of life.

www.ingramcontent.com/pod-product-compliance
Lightning Source LLC
Chambersburg PA
CBHW022133280326
41933CB00007B/673